Sex Positions

Sex Skills He Cannot Resist.

Make Him Beg for More!

information in question by the reader will render any resulting actions solely under their purview. There are no scenarios in which the publisher or the original author of this work can be in any fashion deemed liable for any hardship or damages that may befall them after undertaking information described herein.

Additionally, the information in the following pages is intended only for informational purposes and should thus be thought of as universal. As befitting its nature, it is presented without assurance regarding its prolonged validity or interim quality. Trademarks that are mentioned are done without written consent and can in no way be considered an endorsement from the trademark holder.

Table of Contents

Introduction

I want to extend to you, dear reader, my greatest gratitude for taking the time to purchase this book. Without you, my work would be aimless. Thank you for giving it a purpose.

In this carefully crafted book, you will find an abundance of information on how to pleasure your man better, and more rigorously than you ever thought possible! Topics which are covered range anywhere from the root elements of seduction, to the pinnacle of the male orgasm. Sex is a timeless act of passion, and over the generations, many misconceived notions surrounding the roles of both genders have emerged. A portion of this text will examine this as well.

It is crucial to understand the special aspects to your partner's reproductive system to develop better practices to use in fueling his desire. Renowned tips and tricks concerning: foreplay, fetishes, oral sex, as well as insight on sex positions, are all covered herein.

While this book is meant to be educational and enrich your pre-existing understanding of these concepts, it is by no means an exhaustive or all-in-one resource; as there are hundreds of other books, blogs, web articles, and testimonials that cover these topics, as well as many others. In respect to that, I'd like to thank you once again for choosing this book as your preferred go-to for information! Every effort was made to ensure that the text inside is as accurate and complete as possible. Enjoy the journey!

Chapter 1:
Why Seduce Him?

Just like the timeless adage which suggests a farmer will reap what he sows in his planting field, a great relationship is built from the roots up. And if we were to visualize love as a seed that grows over time, we would have to accredit the art of seduction as the foundation for which the rest is built upon. Seduction, perhaps one of the most elusive aspects in the romance department, is the adhesive component that layers a relationship with excitement from the beginning, and holds it together when external factors may otherwise threaten to tear it down later in its course. So why then, does that invigorating feeling we experienced the first time he bought into our game of cat and mouse seem to fade into a dull, monotonous rhythm of predictability? How do we make every episode of sex feel as unparalleled as that *very* first time each and every time? The key ladies, lies in how we bait our partners. And to improve how we're playing the game, it is important that we first dive into some of the psychology behind how attraction works from the opposite perspective.

Attraction

What were the thoughts running through our mind that afternoon we were sitting in the dine-in section of Noodles

& Company, and in strutted that big, brawny, cowboy with the chest descended from the gods? Oh, how hot it suddenly feels as we sat up a bit straighter, pushing our bosom together to give our breast that nice firm look, and smiling so obviously that our best friend turns around simultaneously to get a glimpse of the view that's abruptly captured our attention. How ecstatic it felt as together, we worked up that plot from the seats of our booth to lure him in and get his number. And the thrill when it succeeded! How about a few days later when he so awkwardly asked you out, and the rush of endorphins that accompanied the first date: Tuscan Italian followed by a moonlit walk through the park. Remember those little push pull tactics that seemed to always leave him wanting more? Everything seemed so perfect. So what happened?

It's no secret that the first time we meet a member of the opposite sex whom we are attracted to, we may be experiencing many different emotions. Instinctively, we try to use every tool at our disposal to ensure that we get them to reciprocate the same feelings back at us. Thus, seduction is born. We play the game and we play it professionally. We win our prize. And then naturally over time, the trophy starts to lose its shine. The way which we first viewed him begins to lose significance. We find ourselves desiring to spice things up with another who will keep things interesting. And much to our disdain, we've already noticed little things that signify our partner is seeking to do the same (but he thought he was being so sneaky)!

Although it may be disheartening to hear, this is completely normally. As a relationship progresses, both parties can begin to fall victim to emotional neglect. What once seemed special now seems expendable. And expendable doesn't seem worth fighting for does it? But that's the thing: it is worth fighting for. The grass will always be greener on the other side, and we need to keep that in mind as we consider our next move. Now is not the time to throw in the towel. It's high time to get the creative juices flowing again, and restore the romance to its former glory. And to do that, we need to incorporate some of the same techniques that got the candle burning in the first place.

Tension

We oftentimes will hear it said that conflict can be healthy in a relationship to a certain degree. And at the foundation of conflict is tension. Creating tension repeatedly is absolutely vital to the continued survival of a strong sex life and overall relationship with your partner. Because tension is correlated closely to our emotions, it's bound to release physically sooner or later. Our goal is to establish that *need* to release continuously by seducing our partner habitually and frequently. In this way, we keep our sex lives feeling fresh and the bond between us and our partner remains strong.

Trust

Just as it's crucial to keep a consistent level of tension built up in a relationship, it is also important that we keep it real with the man in our life, and prove to him continuously that we are the same woman he woed from the get go, and that the personality he fell for wasn't simply a false shroud we donned to win his interest. We want him to feel good whenever possible, and if we suddenly start acting like a different person, it's bound to backfire on the general level of attraction he has for us as well.

Chapter 2:
Common Mistakes Women Make In
Sex

Let's be honest with ourselves ladies. As much as we'd love to lay the blame on our male counterparts for everything as we analyze our sex life, we aren't completely eradicated of blame. In fact, it may come as somewhat of a shocker that the little entitlements we associate with our sex lives are oftentimes the same things that turn him off and originate the feeling of distance that begins to come between our tender feelings. In this section, we're going to go over a few of the biggest no-no's when it comes to motivating his sex drive. You can use this insight the next time you get in the sack to empower his libido with newfound vigor and enthusiasm!

Being Unresponsive

Regarding "the sack", please ladies, when having intercourse don't just lay there as if you quite literally are one! How eager do you really think he's going to be to give it to you on a regular basis if he anticipates coming home to have sex with little more than a living corpse after a hard day's work? Take a tip from the R. Kelly song and mix up the location a bit. A steamy encounter in the kitchen, on the sofa, or even the living room recliner are sure to leave him overjoyed and break up the somber routine in the bedroom.

Playing Mommy Too Literally

Childbirth is truly a marvelous phenomenon. But having kids alone doesn't justify trading in sexy for stagnant! Show him that you still value the mysterious and primal aspect of a sexual encounter. Don't allow your sex life to become a chore that gets procrastinated indefinitely and then performed as quickly as possible (but hopefully not too quickly) to get it over with. Spend some time keeping things interesting by leading a trail of clues to the bedroom, subtly tease him over dinner, and dress in clothing that makes you feel good and reveals just enough to make his imagination run wild as he goes about his daily agenda. In short, it's okay to stay sexy. Remember, you're a mother, not a grandmother yet!

Be What You Were Born To Be

In today's society, women play a bigger role than ever. Sometime we dismiss the traditional housewife persona in favor of playing the new and improved Ms. Congeniality of Wall Street. And why shouldn't we? After all, a woman can do any task just as well as a man (and exceed them in many circumstances!). With that being said, we still need to recognize when it's an appropriate time to whip off the work blouse and whip out the lingerie. You are a woman and you are beautiful. Don't neglect to bedazzle with your femininity!

Fear of Letting Lose

With the many mixed messages in today's world concerning the do's and don'ts of womanhood, it's not surprising that many of us are afraid that if we allow ourselves to appear lewd between the sheets, it will correspond to him developing a belief that we are slutty or some other stereotype with negative connotations. Due to this belief, we may abstain from providing him with the full amount of pleasure we're capable of giving. Allow me to invalidate this belief; as countless men have admitted to speaking admirably about the lady-turned freak between the sheets to their friends and co-workers. Remember, men have wild imaginations! Fulfill his fantasy by being a naughty girl. "Dirty" should definitely **not** be disregarded during sex.

Not Properly Communicating

Most men are far from adept in the department of mind reading, and similarly, you can't assume that he's registering those little hints you're throwing him while he's panting away going down on you and you're wondering what you're currently missing on the Starz channel. Of course, there's no need to be a Debbie Downer and completely kill the vibe either! Consider speaking up more frequently when he's trying something that clearly isn't working for you. This is to allow him to know it's time to pull another rabbit out of the hat. On the contrary, **do** provide him with positive encouragement through both your verbal and nonverbal body languages when he's doing a stellar job at performing.

Displaying Insecurities Toward Other Women

Openly showing feelings of inferiority toward other members of our gender is never a good look. Honey, don't forget there's a whole sea of fish out there but you're the only one he gets to call his catch. Take pride in yourself, and dominate his body!

You Aren't Giving Fellatio

For some couples, the realm of oral sex is a sensitive topic. Some women find it to be unsophisticated, distastefully, or just downright gross. That's okay, but don't assume that the situation is going to remedy itself automatically. Talk to him about his desires, and substitute other methods of erotic stimulation if necessary. To coin a phrase an old friend of mine used to say, "There's more than one way to skin a cat."

Chapter 3:
Fantasies

When exploring the vast realm of sexual fantasy and stimulation for the first time, it's relatively easy to conjure up images of bondage and submissive behavior; such as something we would witness in the popular film 50 Shades of Grey. And while pain and pleasure undoubtedly are a superb concoction to set the tone for any erotic pipe-dream, allow me to reassure you ladies that it doesn't require an extended weekend getaway in a secluded penthouse apartment to leave your man breathless. In fact, according to the Business Insider, a recent survey conducted in Quebec showed that when men think about sex, at least five of the reoccurring fantasies involve the same scenarios that we imagine. Among these are thoughts about:

> Having sex with someone who isn't our partner

> Having sex in strange locations

> Having sex in a romantic location

> Masturbating our partner

> Perverse methods of oral sex

The truth is, when formulating a plan to fulfill all of our partner's dirty little daydreams in real life, we don't need to spend large amounts of money acquiring chains, whips, and toys for foreplay (although that certainly is an option as well). The typical structure for male sex fantasies can be divided into two categories: the first one involves basic core elements that they can pull from memory any time that suits them. The second is more subjective to the world around them; what catches their attention in public or on television, and how they could manipulate it into a steamy sexcapade. We can use this knowledge to our advantage by utilizing the mentioned core elements, and improvise other creative ways to spice up the scene as we go along. The following are a few great concepts to you can customize to make your own, that are sure to get some kinky chemistry flowing between the two of you:

Dominance

Contrary to the customary belief that dominant sex requires a lot of fancy equipment, there are actually two distinct aspects to asserting dominance in the bedroom: physical and verbal. Let's take a few moments to examine both respectively:

Physicality

Deviating from your traditional positions during intercourse is perhaps the first and most obvious remedy to cut the monotony out of your sex and make things more interesting. One suggestion would be to straddle him like a cowgirl while he sits on a chair. This severely limits his mobility, while also shifting power over the situation into your hands.

Playing Games

Another simple solution to infuse yourself as the dominant role during sex is to introduce some games into the routine. You might for example, let him know that you're about to make all of his wildest fantasies happen and the only condition is that he can't so much as make a sound, grunt, or mumble whilst you please him. You can take this even further by punishing him with spanks any time your ground-rule is broken.

It goes without saying that teasing a tied up hunk is hot! Ask him prior to your next play date if he would be interested in experimenting with techniques involving restraints and bondage, and pick up the required materials ahead of time.

Verbal Dominance

Effectively enforcing verbal domination over your partner is best done by laying a foundation upon which you then gradually rev up into more blunt and stringent commands. An example of putting this method into action would be to begin asking him to do tasks for you around the house on Monday. By Wednesday, you remove the conditional language and make a statement telling him what he is **going** to do versus what he wants to do. After observing his compliance at this phase, you move onto the sex specifically. By this point, you would have removed any lavishness to your requests and be tossing in more and more extremities; telling him he isn't allowed to come until you say so and other things of that nature.

Submission

You may also be intrigued by the idea of shifting the power to the opposite end of the spectrum; that is, you would be assuming the role of submissive to his bidding during sex. Similar to the scenario when you were the dominant, the demands he may be impressing onto you as his submissive more often than not will extend beyond the bedroom. Because of this, it is of the utmost importance that you discuss the details and your individual level of comfort with what you're about to attempt before putting it into action to avoid things going too far and crossing over the abuse threshold. Alternatively, an option for ensuring safe implementation of the games is to play the "bottom". Essentially, a bottom receives the same level of direction and discipline as a submissive, but with a mutual understanding that the role is temporary and exclusive only to certain areas of the residence.

Acting the Part

It's fairly typical to witness the submissive, or bottom, as the individual who is blindfolded, gagged, or otherwise restricted during the games. Depending on the preferences of your party, you might allow him to have generous privileges in the anal category, or kick things off by giving him a lengthy blow job to smooth the transition into the role of inferiority. He might require you to ask for permission prior to performing certain actions, or give you a name that you must refer to him by for the tenure of your session.

Safe Words

While it's certainly commendable that you're stepping out of your comfort zone and cranking up the notch on your sex life in the first place, it's also quite understandable that you may have a certain degree of fear and reluctance accompanying this new world of sexual experimentation. To that extent, it's time to unveil "safe words." Safe words should be easy to recall under pressure, and signify that it's time for him to let up on the game and snap back to reality so that the pair of you can address the circumstance that's creating the unwarranted discomfort. If you do not feel like choosing your own safe words, another option is to use the stoplight system, which is essentially a model that mirrors a traffic light. For instance, saying "green" would beckon your partner to go ahead, yellow would mean let off the gas (metaphorically speaking), and red would mean he needs to call it quits.

Duality

Keep in mind that nothing need be black and white when it comes to implementing rules. You could both take turns experimenting with the separate roles to broaden your horizons to the various possibilities available at your disposal. A person who trades between being the submissive and the dominant is generally referred to as the "switch." Above all, remember that although bondage can initially seem a bit bizarre, it should never be a frightening experience. By keeping a proper line of communication and honesty open between yourself and your partner, you may surprisingly find that this type of sex brings you closer together than ever before!

Explicit Oral Sex

When it comes to the kind of fantasies that men think about, research has unanimously shown that the broadest and most common theme that comes into play involves us women behaving badly in ways that we would normally never consent to. If you're the type who finds it more than a little un-lady like to go down on him, doing just that could potentially be your best and most effort-effective solution to literally blow his mind! In the early 2000's, there was a notable song lyric in which the artist proclaimed he "loved having sex, but he'd rather get some head." And when it comes to making our men melt in the palm of our hand, few phrases could be truer.

Role Playing

Who doesn't like dressing up for fun? Having an opportunity to pretend to be somebody else (and for a justifiable purpose!) during sex is an extremely renowned and timeless way to experience the thrill of having multiple partners while remaining faithful and enthusiastic in a relationship. For an alpha male, this could be a unique way to create an illusion of authority and power over a lesser, attractive female subject. Or, feel free to make your own character variants and adjust turn the tables as you see fit using some of the previously discussed fantasies. The sky's truly the limit here. If you find yourself running short on ideas, here are some propositions to lay the groundwork for your role-play:

- ➢ Fireman

- ➢ Teacher/Student

- ➢ Good Cop/Bad Cop

- ➢ G.I. Joe & Jane

- ➢ Naughty Nurse

Exhibitionism

I had a guy friend several years back who used to confide in me quite openly in regards to his sex life. He admitted once that among the items on his bucket list of "dirty deeds," was to have sex inside of the toilet stall of a shopping mall during business hours. He went on to explain how, in his opinion, the prospect of being walked in on in conjunction with the filthy environment of a public restroom, was a delightful overload for his mind to soak up whenever he pondered it.

Not surprisingly, confessions akin to this have been made by a large number in the male population. It would almost seem as though one could conclude that any act going directly against the conventional order of things, or acceptable mannerisms of society, is fair play for a sexually arousing fantasy. With that awareness in mind, do be sure to execute caution if you choose to dive into this area of enlightenment ladies, as I'm sure you do not need to be informed about the extensive legal fines and penalties that can result from being caught indecently exposed in the wrong setting.

Chapter 4:
Foreplay (Stimulate The Mind Before The Body)

The Importance of Taking Your Time

Although it could be argued that quick sex is still better than no sex, ideally sex should never be rushed, and adequate time should be allowed for foreplay at the initiation of a good ole' romp in the sheets. Evidence has shown that both genders experience a more fulfilling orgasm during their respective culminations when stimulation occurred prior to intercourse. It's also important to note that by spending more time focusing on becoming aroused, you'll also be spending considerably more time with him performing "the act" itself on a grander scale. Of course, this matters because with the amount of stresses and commitments already plopped into our everyday lives, it's likely seldom you're able to dedicate much time, if any, to focus solely on each other and shut out the distractions of the outside world. By allowing ample time for bodily pleasure, you'll not only feel more refreshed after sex, but also be doing your relationship a big favor in the department of mutual good feelings to be had all around; both inside and outside of the bedroom.

Techniques That Will Leave Him Speechless

Showcase The Goods

That's right. Your biggest asset is the one your momma gave you: that beautiful body with the voluptuous curves. Start by giving him a striptease and be sure to caress all the sweet spots to get his imagination going. To further enhance the torment for him, consider strapping his arms to the bedposts, or tying him up in front of a mirror while you do a suggestive little dance, letting your outer garments fall to the floor. Make sure you do everything unbearably slow so that by the time you move onto the next phase, he can no longer contain himself from ferociously groping you in all the right areas.

Touch Him Generously

I assume that when you were young you knew at least a handful of kids who were more ticklish than others. Recall how you could sneak up on them and drive them to the brink of wetting their pants simply by using your hands under their armpits. Now apply that same mischievousness with an R-rated twist and you'll be well on your way to giving your partner the best sex he's ever had! Men require a thorough amount of hands on stimulation to fully maximize their arousal, and not just in the obvious location down under. Tell him to lay face down on his stomach while you lay your naked body over his back side and massage his ass, pinch his sides, and caress his shoulder blades. Next, flip him over and work his front side from the top down; avoiding the sweet spot until the last possible moment to build up his anticipation!

Just Breathe

A lot can be accomplished with an alternating flux of hot and cool air when it comes to getting him worked up. Akin to touching, it's recommended that you begin somewhere opposite his package, such as his neck. Let your lips hover in place momentarily, then slowly exhale of warm air over that region. Kiss your way down to his nipples and give them a few tender licks. Follow up with blowing a couple rapid spurts of cool air on top. The contrasting temperature will spike his senses in a most agonizingly pleasurable manner. Continue the pattern as you arrive at his penis. You don't have to go licking away yet, but position your lips the same way in which you'd blow out a scented candle and let some more cold air off over his tip. By the time you've finished, he will practically be begging to have your body.

So You Like to Play Rough?

By their very nature, men generally take a more hands on approach to tasks than their female counterparts. The bedroom is no exception here, and being the strong man that he is, your partner is probably contributing the majority of forceful action into the fray. However, given the choice, most men would prefer his woman take the wheel every now and then and exert some muscle into the mix. He'll have no problem with you asserting him in this manner, as it registers in his mind as being challenged for control and he almost instinctively finds this to be a sexy attribute. In these circumstances, it's perfectly okay to step outside the box and get more aggressive. Run your hands down his back, and sink your nails in just far enough to make an impression as you nibble on his lower lip. Show him whose boss; when he attempts to go down on you, push him over on his back and revert him to the receiving end of the spectrum. Believe me, he will welcome the surprise!

Leave Him Hanging

Now; just as he's reaching the apex of intensity, it's time to put the icing on the cake with a classic bait and switch. The entire area from his thighs to genitals is a kind of "bullseye" of the nerves, so draw an invisible circle around the area and keep playing the hot/cold game with your mouth. Observe his body language for indicators that he is about to bust, then recede enough to allow him to recover. The ball is in your court at this point (or should I say balls plural)?

Props

Here, I've taken the liberty of including a list of toys the consensus of males have said are "must have's," as well as a list that's best to be avoided:

Yes Please

> ➤ Lipstick

> ➤ Wigs

> ➤ Fishnet socks

> ➤ Polaroid Cameras

No Thankyou

> ➤ High Heels

> ➤ Candle Wax

> ➤ Chocolate syrup

> ➤ Lotion

Alternative Considerations

It may or may not have already occurred to you, but with the already vast menagerie of tools available to assist you with his arousal, foreplay doesn't really have to begin in bed whatsoever. Here are a few more ideas to help you diversify your pre-game:

Going Clubbing

Even if the vibrancy of your current sex life has dropped to all-time lows, a night out on the town is sure to change that. The atmosphere of nearly any electronic dance club is riddled with suggestive vibes and sensually pleasing music. He'll have a hard time abstaining from an erection while you're preoccupied grinding on his entire lower-half!

Take A Couples Bath

If you're both in the mood for something a bit more low-key, consider taking a nice, hot, bath together to unwind from a long day. Enter wearing a see-through, revealing garment, and gradually accelerate the pace by fondling each other until you deem that it's time to take it off. A bath is a practical way to reap the benefits of foreplay with minimal effort involved for both of you.

Let's Talk About Sexting

For some steamy entertainment, bust out the disposable camera and let him go to town on the photo reel. Alternatively, you may want to sext him some exclusive pictures of yourself while both of you are apart during the day, to get excited well in advance. Regardless of the type of camera you decide to go with, it's advised that you discard the photos by the end of your sexual encounter, so as to limit any potential data leaks of your birthday suit bonanza.

Watching Porn Isn't Trashy

"Netflix n' Chill" isn't the only way to get fired up watching TV together. As long as there isn't any objection for personal reasons, getting comfortable in front of a porn-flick actually has a demonstrated effect of bringing relationships closer. Not to mention it'll hopefully teach you both a few new tricks of the trade along the way.

Chapter 5:
Oral Sex (Make His Legs Turn To Jelly!)

Do you recall that summer occasion years ago when you attended a bonfire at the lake cabin of your middle-school's head cheerleader. By half past midnight, everybody was busy making out or cuddling with their new squeeze. You had spent the afternoon bonding with that cute boy wearing the skater-branded swim trunks and brandishing that forearm tattoo that suggested from the beginning that he was well accustomed to breaking a few rules. While the rest of your friends and acquaintances were occupied, the two of you snuck off to the big willow tree on the edge of the front lawn, where he chivalrously splayed out his hoodie like a makeshift blanket. The next thing you knew, you were sprawled over each other kissing with the fiery passion of summer romance as the sound of distant fireworks crackled through the night air. After several minutes, the smacking turned into groping, and the groping led to the top portion of your polka-dotted two-piece suddenly visible in the grass next to your now half naked bodies. He was already nearly finished with getting the belt unfastened on his jeans, and hastily unbuttoning his fly. When completed, his semi-erect penis was protruding thru the opening like a small serpent and he was gesturing for you to get your face down there. Hardly a quarter of the way into your teenage years at the time, you weren't expecting this request, and hesitantly you asked him if it was possible to get pregnant by mistakenly swallowing. He seemed to be mockingly laughing at you as he quickly dissuaded your concern and once again beckoned for your mouth on his crotch. You reluctantly complied. When he came and it was over, he stood up, re-fastened his studded belt and walked away without so much as a glance back over his shoulder. You remember sitting there replaying the scene to yourself over and over. Did you do something wrong? Did he think you were "bad" at giving oral?

Fortunately, as you got older and wiser, you discovered that he was just an asshole and it was time to let bygones be bygones. But as I'm sure you've had at least a handful of one-night stands in the years between your youth and womanhood, you've undoubtedly been on both the giving and receiving end of oral in numerous circumstances. Why is oral so desired by both sexes as a warm-up to intercourse? Is there any significance to having it from a medical standpoint? Or is it simply another fantasy of the flesh we yearn to have fulfilled? Let's take a look:

How Have Cunnilingus And Fellatio Evolved?

As far as any historic evidence may suggest, humans have been partaking in oral sex for as long as they've been partaking in standard intercourse. So, that means quite literally: from genesis. Although case studies specific to humans are somewhat limited (let's be honest not everybody is comfortable with allowing bystanders to film the act) data collected from observing bats has shown that performing fellatio can make them last longer during intercourse. Additionally, the lubrication provided from the female bats may increase the overall level of comfort during penetration. As far as cunnilingus goes, males who participated in surveys reported that they were more likely to go down on their partner if they believed that she was attractive to other men, in attempt to keep her faithful. The vast majority of women would agree that being the recipient of good cunnilingus causes them to have a heightened orgasm by the time the climax during regular intercourse, and helps compensate for what might otherwise be mediocre sex. A key point that remains here however is that the presence or absence of oral sex is rarely the sole culprit at fault when cheating is at stake. Rather, it's all about doing your duty to ensure your partner is enjoying themselves as a whole, and finding out what could be done differently if that isn't the case.

The Bottom Line

I'll wrap up this segment by stating that while the precise origin of both fellatio and cunnilingus are open to discussion, we can conclude that at the most primitive level, the primary function of intercourse is still procreation of life, whereas oral sex is a forerunner with the main purpose of providing added lubrication and stimulation. Now that I've covered the more mundane snippets of information, let's get onto the juicy part where I'll discuss some of the best practices to teach you how to pleasure your mate like a porn-star; and as the chapter title hinted: turn his legs to jelly!

To become better at anything, practice makes it perfect. In the category of giving your partner fellatio, that saying holds true as ever. If you do happen to be somewhat inexperienced when it comes to this, my first recommendation is that you start by picking up a box of pop-sickles, bananas, or any other lengthy edible item that resembles the likeness of his cock, and spend some of your free time getting becoming familiar with the motion. That may sound slightly corny, but trust me, although I'm confident that your partner has enough tact not to criticize you while you're trying to please him, one thing you **do not** want to get in the habit of doing is giving a blowjob full of teeth. Refine your technique using only your lips and slowly introduce your tongue along the side of the shaft.

Practice the art of "rimming," which involves bringing your mouth to the tip and letting it slide back to the point where it connects to the shaft while keeping your lips pursed together in a round fashion. Once you've mastered that, you should be well equipped to move onto your true test subject without doing any harm. You would still do well to ask for, and implement his feedback once you're through (mid-sex might not be the most optimal time for conversation) to continue to develop and improve your technique in a manner that tailors to his individual needs. As a general overview, here are some hot tips to making your next encounter a very memorable occurrence:

Let Me See Your Hands

This one is subjective to the individual. However, most of the time, using your hand and your mouth simultaneously will enhance the experience for your man. Experiment with different ranges of motion suited to his needs. Try stroking him with a firm grasp, bringing your hand all the way over the top of his head (his southernmost head!) with each upward repetition of the movement. Brace yourself, and allow him to gag you every so often; bringing your mouth all the way down to his package and holding in place for a few seconds before pulling back out. Periodically fondle his scrotum while sucking to hit him with an erotic double-whammy!

Setting The Tone

When using your mouth, don't feel like you're strictly limited to the same sucking motion. Oftentimes as women, we feel insecure with completely letting ourselves run wild during sex for fear of how it will be received. But that's precisely what can make the difference between giving **good** head and giving **great** head. Alternate the sucking with licking. Again, his entire genital territory is your play place here so go roaming wherever you'd like. Look into his eyes when you transit into doing something new to see how he's handling it. Listen for his moans and compliments, as this will also cue you on when to work him more rapidly.

Halt His Flow Right In Its Tracks!

This part can sometimes be a bit tricky and create a conundrum. Should you spit, swallow, or finish him off with your hand and take his load right into your palm? Ladies, the best way to make your decision here is to think to yourself how would you feel if you were in his shoes at this very moment? If he made abrupt changes to his trajectory, wouldn't it diminish your climax? The answer is probably yes. Therefore, the good answer here is to do whatever comes naturally for you. Although some men find it quite flattering (and impressive) when a woman swallows his seed, I'm aware that not everybody reading this will find that to be feasible. If you do choose to swallow, it might not be a bad idea to keep an old towel nearby, just in case it decides to come back out; preferably voluntarily!

As you build up with more experience with your partner, you may have better grasp at his climax timings and more familiar with his body cues prior his climax. This can give you sufficient time to stroke him with your hands and allow his seeds to cum on your bosoms or face. Many men find it really arousing and accomplished this way! Make him feel that he's on top of the world!

Other Things To Try

The Edging Technique

More or less exactly what the heading implies. The goal is to bring him right up to the "edge" of his climax and back off before he has a chance to go over the top. This typically will result in him having a more powerful and satisfying **finale** further along when he absolutely can't hold out any longer.

Reciprocating The Sounds of Love

I mean c'mon right? Why not at least show him you're enjoying the moment as much as he is (well maybe not **quite** as much). Throw in some moans to accompany his own while still keeping a mouthful of his privates. As mentioned previously, keep the lingo brief to allow him to become fully immersed in the ecstasy; but don't hesitate to ask him if he likes it as you get fancy down there (he will).

Get It Wet

The more the merrier when it comes to moisture. Providing additional saliva will only add to his state of stimulation. If you're running into dry mouth issues, consider sucking on a breath-mint before you get started as has proven to be beneficial in getting the waterworks going in our salivary glands. Consider saturating his shaft with coconut oil in lieu of spit for a great taste!

Sprays

If you've noticed that your gag reflex is creating a blockade in this department, there are specialty sprays manufactured specifically for oral sex. You won't find any of them to be as strong as a prescription medication for sore throat per say, but it should serve as a viable solution to help you go longer than you typically could before hitting a wall.

Can Too Much of A Good Thing Be Bad?

The short answer here is yes. Everything I've talked about so far has revolved around maximizing his induced level of pleasure. And ultimately that's what we're after. But let's think about it for a minute. From the male perspective, if we were to pack our boyfriend or husband a piece of cake every day to take along with his lunch to work, there would more than likely come a point where he gets tired of it; or at the very least, learns to rely on it being there so much that it ceases to be a treat to look forward too. Following that same logic, I wouldn't give my boyfriend or husband a BJ more often than is reasonably deserved. As a rule of thumb, I'd say about once per week is sufficient, or to mark a special occasion where you deem he deserves to be rewarded. This will prevent him developing dependence or other unrealistic expectations.

So, You Come Here Often?

If you've been reading this book from the beginning, you're going to recognize that this next pointer borrows several characteristics from exhibitionism (discussed in an earlier chapter on male sex fantasies). Obviously, when we have oral sex, ninety-five percent of the time we'll be doing it in the bedroom. But don't segregate yourself to the master suite exclusively, or I can assure you that you're going to be missing out on tapping into a whole other box of kinky magic. Sure, you could give him head in other rooms of the household, but can you imagine the look on his face if you were to pull him aside at the company Christmas party, in the garden, or even a secluded area at the beach, and blow him? I'm by no means suggesting you break any laws to get your kicks, and just like I discussed on the topic of exhibitionism; you will need to be wary of that. Nevertheless, I hope it has at least broadened your horizons as to what's possible in regards to this topic.

All About Anilingus

Thus far, my tips on oral sex have revolved around the penis and corresponding tissue only. There is however, another, less mainstream (but not lesser by any means!) method of activating vast amounts of pleasure known as anilingus. There is a rough section of skin that sits just behind his testicles called the *perineum*. In a nutshell (no pun intended) anilingus involves licking this area all around the same manner in which you would give him a sloppy BJ. Some guys are really into it, while others find it repulsive. Therefore, this is one of those instances where it's vital to have a conversation with him well ahead of time to determine which group he falls into.

What's The Word?

For the record, the word anilingus is interchangeable with **analingus** and may be referred to as such. Regardless of the phonetic manipulation, both describe the same thing. Common slang may also allude to the phrase "tossing the salad" when discussing the act.

In Preparation

Due to the large amount of bacteria that breed in and around the rectum, it is pertinent that proper hygiene is adhered to by both you and him prior to the commencement of anilingus. Make him take a shower and shave as much hair as possible away from the area. Verify that he's been checked for, and is free of sexually transmitted diseases prior to proceeding.

Breaking Down The Techniques

Toothy Fruity

Here's a big dissimilarity to giving head from the front side: the teeth aren't shunned upon here. Not surprising, gently raking your teeth across his anus is the propellant factor for getting him off here. As always, keep it gentle. Sinking your fangs in probably wouldn't feel or taste very good in this situation!

Up Down & All Around

Easiest of the bunch, during this technique, your tongue will remain on outside of his body at all times. All you need to do is ready a plethora of saliva, make like a lizard and start licking to the sides, in a circle, or any combination between. The focus should primarily be on the anus itself, although it's fine to deviate slightly to the skin immediately surrounding it.

Just A Little Poke

Successive to the "up, down, and all around" technique, this one gets more personal. As in, you're going to tighten the muscles in your tongue, and using the point, begin thrusting in and out of his rectum. You won't be able to make it in further than approximately a half-inch, so don't be overly concerned with encountering any nasty surprises during penetration.

Poopey Smooches

Eventually, all that tongue action is going to wear you out; and that's when kissing comes into play. Keeping your lips as moist as possible, begin succulently pressing to his rectum and let your tongue have a few rounds on the sideline.

Alternative Options

The Power of Your Finger

While allowing your tongue a few well deserved moments of respite from the action, you can insert your finger into his anus to stimulate his prostate and other interior rectal components. Because your finger is stronger than your tongue, it also won't cramp up so easily.

Scratch Those Cheeks

A standalone semi-technique in itself; this is precisely what it sounds like. Although this only provides a minor amount of stimulation alone, paired with your tongue, this technique is bound to feel great to him.

Assume The Position

Pay special heed the following descriptions, as the following positions for performing anilingus are designed to keep his ass cheeks spread as far apart as possible to help you comfortably prevail and not feel like you're desperately surfacing for air by the time you're finished:

Bend Over And Touch Your...Ankles

I hope he's been taking tips from you when you do those Pilates in the living room, because this one requires some flexibility on his part. Simply tell him to bend over and grab the front of his ankles while you get on your knees from behind, and go to town using your technique of choice.

Ankle Touching While Lying Prone

There isn't much difference between the standard ankle-grab and this variation. The main purpose of doing it this way is to get his arms out of the way so that you can add in a hand-job while tossing the salad synchronously. This would also be easier for him to accomplish the same movement if he's flunking on flexibility.

The Low Down On Deep-Throating

According to Kinkly.com, the explicit phenomenon of deep-throating originated it's hype from a 1972 porno in which a young women is taken advantage of by her doctor; who informs her that her clitoris is lodged at the back of her throat, and manipulates her into inhaling his entire salami, as well as that of several cohorts.

Domesticating Your Gag

Previously in this chapter, I touched on the topic of practice being crucial to giving a good blowjob. We're going to take that into slightly more intermediate territory here when talking about how to immunize your gag-reflex for good; known as *desensitization*. Below, I'm going to outline a step by step method with proven results in managing this. Master this procedure, and move onto your man with the confidence of a professional!

Desensitization In Ten Steps

1) Obtain a dildo, banana, or other oblong item.

2) Stick it in your mouth, and gradually push it back toward the back of your esophagus.

3) When you feel that it is beginning to come on, suppress your gag reflex.

4) Breathe through your nose while maintaining diligent concentration. This is rather difficult, but keeping practicing and don't give up!

5) Hold the item in place at the back of your throat for several seconds without moving it.

6) Do this a few times each day for an entire week. Notice how as the week progresses, your gag becomes less and less prominent during practice sessions.

7) As the weeks continue, you'll notice your gag reflex is becoming next to non-existent. At this point, it's time to start adding in movement of the object; into and out of your mouth to mimic what his penis will be doing.

8) At first this will spur the vomit sensation you experienced when you first began training your gag reflex. It's important that you relax and don't

become too discouraged even if your throat is convulsing.

9) When you've practiced this intermediate phase for a few more weeks, you should be relatively at ease with moving the object in and out of your mouth without falling victim to gagging any longer.

10) Finally, it's time for the real deal!

I'm just going to reiterate that this **is** the most proven method of learning to contain your gag reflex. Likewise, it's the most cost effective as the only thing you need is a single penis-shaped prop, and some commitment.

Chapter 6:
The Best Sex Positions
No Man Can Resist

Here at last we've arrived at the headlining exhibit of our sexual adventure, appropriately named: the best sex positions from a male perspective. To recap thus far, we've discussed the purpose of getting your partner excited during flirtatious interactions, mistakes that most women take for granted related to their part in sex, as well as some thematic male sex fantasies. We've provided you with some ideas to use during foreplay, and a descriptive version of giving him the best blowjob of his life, directly preceding this section.

Now comes the moment you've been waiting for (and maybe your entire motivation for picking up this book in the first place)! So please set aside your notes on the appetizers, because now you are going to be shown how to serve him the main course.

- *The following resembles data accumulated from thousands of men over a recent period of time, and aren't listed in any particular order. They are not provided with the intent of implying that your specific partner will find them preferential to the many other erotic poses out there; but rather, based on the majority of reports.*

7 Nights In Heaven: The Top Choices of Sex Positions For Men

The Reverse Cowgirl

While your man lies down on his back, straddle him; either by keeping your knees flush to the bed, or squatting with feet flat on the mattress. Brace yourself by putting your arms on his thighs or reaching backward and caressing his chest as you commence movement. Utilize either up and down motions, or whirl your hips as he thrusts to fully activate your G-Spot as he goes. Feel free to get your own hand dirty, since you'll have full access and control from up here.

As mentioned previously, guys love a woman who takes the driver's seat! Among other benefits of "the cowgirl" is the view he gets of your entire backside while he goes at it. Since this position leaves you with a lot of space to improvise, try playing with his balls to make him moan even harder. Just be sure not to lean too far in any direction throughout the thrusting. After all, his pogo-stick isn't made of plastic.

Stay Standing

Quickie compatible and custom fitted to his manhood, this position might not be what you'd consider a five-star experience, but then again, this is for his party, we're just here to help with the setup. Besides he'll love getting an all in one bicep workout as he balances your body against the wall!

Get Your Bounce Around On Top

This time, instead of facing away from him as demonstrated in "the reverse cowgirl," you are going to allow him to grab the goody-bags as we bounce around above him. It should be noted that this is not an occasion that constitutes dimming the lights! Let him take in all the eye-candy his heart desires.

Missionary

Are you at all shocked to learn that the notorious "69" made one of his top spots on the bedroom bucket-list? Intimate yet steamy, you'll be able to set the pace congruently; while keeping eyes locked on each other. Act as his road map and pull his hips closer when desiring a deeper thrust. You can communicate almost entirely using your body when things are this "up close and personal." Additionally, you can alleviate the lifeless stereotype of the missionary position by throwing these suggestions into the mix:

- You Deserve A Spanking

Show him your approval by giving him a firm and unexpected swat!

- Pillow Pants

A number of specialists have suggested that elevating your butt into a heightened position makes deeper penetration possible. Try it! Most couples love this position!

- Kiss, Kiss

You can hold an entire make-out session while your limbs intertwine in this affectionate sex pose.

- Two-In-One

Go ahead and play with yourself in harmony to his rhythm of thrusts. The nipples are just fine as well.

- The Valedictorian

Have him to put your ankles on his shoulders so that your legs make a "V" shape. Both of you still gets to enjoy the eye contact while the deep penetration with G-spots hit makes this even more kinky!

Doggy Style

Giving him permission to enter from behind has traditionally been the trademark of bad girls, so what better way to provide him with a gift that will him keep on giving? He can penetrate deeper from this position, giving an added boost to his ego as well as intensifying the feelings you're already accustomed to during intercourse.

Here are a few ways to take "doggy-style" to even higher extremes:

- Overly Eager?

Instead of completely stripping naked, pull your panties to the side and let the friction work its magic on his cock.

- Go Out Of Bounds

A huge advantage to doggy style is that you have a greater range of diversity when it comes to choosing location. Take a crack at it in the laundry room, over the staircase bannister, or even the kitchen table.

- Nipple Fondness

I would imagine he'll have more fun using your breasts as makeshift handles than your pigtails.

Spooning

When you're in the mood for being cute and lazy, this is the definitive pose. Incorporating a head twist here to kiss him while he works up a sweat. He'll appreciate that he has full access to your body from this vantage point, and you'll appreciate that your hands are free once again to roam wherever you please. Spooning will also keep both of you conveniently in place to take a nice nap afterwards, after all that expenditure of your efforts.

The Lap Dance

The pinnacle pose to satisfy his masculine ego and your stripper side. Pull out a chair, plop him in the hot seat, and climb aboard! Unlike the regular position where you're on top, this one keeps your bodies aligned for the entire duration. You can keep kissing while he rubs your backside up and down and playfully tugs on your hair. He will love the seductive look and irresistible feel of you straddling him with you in control.

The Lazy Man

This position puts you in control and is one of the popular starting positions which continues the sexual transition flow from foreplay arousal. Place pillows behind his back and have him to sit on the bed with legs stretched out straight and crossed. Proceed to sit on his groin area facing him and slowly direct his private in. Just by pressing on the balls of your feet and releasing in a squat thrusting motion, you can raise and lower yourself on his shaft at any speed he pleases. Allow him to embrace you in a tight hug and there is no way he can resist licking your assets in his face.

Interesting Facts About Sex Positions in the Old World

Back in the Middle Ages, the church had a much more prominent influence in everyday life than in modern times. As shocking as it may seem, this reach extended so far, that it even dictated certain regulations that needed to be abided by when having intercourse! For purists, sex was only viewed as a necessity for the survival of the human species. As such, partaking in oral, or anal intercourse was strictly prohibited. Even more so, practicing any sex positions aside from the missionary, was considered a sin because it was believed that a female who took a dominant position during sex conflicted with the naturally hierarchy they were supposed to fit into in society. Imagine having to worry about tedious things like that while you're trying to get off! Punishment for being found in violation of these regulations could be extremely severe for women; including up to three years of forced penance. Interesting to note here is that in that era, men were presumably absolved of any guilt, and did not incur any disciplinary action themselves.

Eventually, a clergyman by the name of Albertus Magnus determined an order of sexual positions which he ranked in order from most acceptable to forbidden. Again it was deemed that the only position which was completely justified was the missionary, whereas the remainder were classified as questionable from a moral standpoint, although no longer "sinful."

Chapter 7:
Climax Move (What To Do When He's Cumming)

The final section of this sex manual of sorts, is going to dive into the unique traits that surround your partner's orgasm, and how you can help ease him along as smoothly as possible to maximize the degree of bliss he experiences leading up to, and upon reaching his "peaking-point."

Establishing A Basic Understanding

When a man looks at something that appeals to him sexually, the arteries located inside of his "vessel" pump blood much more rapidly than normal. The veins contract; retaining the fluid inside of the penis and his sack become taught at the base of the organ.

Now that "he's up," his body involuntarily prepares for the imminent release of semen. He tightens up even more, and his heart rate dramatically increases like somebody running at an intense pace on a treadmill. A transparent fluid may begin to trickle from the tip. The purpose of this fluid is to adjust the chemicals found naturally in his tip, or *urethra,* giving his sperm a greater chance to endure the trials of penetration without dying prematurely. When he comes, he comes in two parts. First, he reaches the "tipping point" where semen begins to rush out and collect at the top of the urethra. From here on out, a series of tiny muscles at the base of his scrotum begin contracting as he ejaculates in short, intense, bursts. Oftentimes, shaking will occur uncontrollably, as he has achieved a state of pleasure overload. Once he's completely spent, his penis will reduce up to half its erectile capacity immediately, he may feel fatigued and low on energy as his body enters a temporary recovery mode. This is the end of the cycle, and he typically will not be able to obtain another erection for at least thirty minutes.

When There's An Issue

Every once in a while, men can run into problematic circumstances with reaching their orgasm. Usually, this is burrowed in something related to an underlying mental barricade, or they've gotten into an unusual or atypical regime of self-masturbation. Temporarily resolving these kinds of issues can usually be relatively easy by using sex toys; whereas a permanent fix will probably require sex therapy. Therapeutic approaches are administered in a way which diminishes the pressure of performance, and puts a heavier emphasis on positive encouragement and centering on the pleasure that encompasses ejaculation.

Getting Him Ready

Flipping The Coin

Now, if I still have your attention (hopefully) after that rant of tedious, but pertinent material, we will continue on ahead. When we digging into the psychology behind the male orgasm, we can think of it like the shot of whiskey he rewards himself with at Friday happy hour proceeding a week from hell at the office. And although it can obviously be said that men reap the same, if not more enjoyment out of their ten seconds in heaven than women do, men, being the egoistic creatures that they are slightly more conditional on when they choose to come. By that I mean that if you were to conduct a poll, the data would conclude that most men will ensure their partner's fulfillment during sex before honing in on their own.

Well, our goal for tonight is to turn the tables on him. You're reading this because you want him to have the time of his life, right? So, we're going to kick off the festivities by putting him at ease from his high standards. There's a couple of ways in which you can go about doing this. The first is you can wait until the sex is already well underway, and drop a line to let him know that tonight is a gift for him and "any way he wants it, that's the way he'll have it." The alternative, and more accredited notion among experts, is that you have him lie down and unwind as you begin your sexual sorcery. The choice is yours, but bear in mind that option two takes the responsibility completely off his shoulders, granting him the ability to fully indulge in his pleasure senses.

Honey, Slow Your Roll

Thanks to the science behind testosterone build-up and male hormones, time is always on the side of us women when it comes to being a tease. Which is precisely what makes this subtle tactic so powerful when used to our advantage. For men, abstinence opens a big vulnerability, and we're going to drag out that sexual deprivation he longs to quench. Make him go several days without any action. Then, earlier on the day you're going to break the dry spell, utilize a handful of the previously outlined strategies regarding foreplay; as they will cross over well into this category. For instance, let him get a glimpse of your breasts while you get dressed, then quickly conceal yourself. Consider sending him a handful of dirty texts when you know he still has seven hours to go on the clock. They will feel like the longest of his life! Especially with all that pent-up tension.

Massage The Perineum

I don't know if anybody would be able to determine the exact reason why such an insignificant quadrant of tissue between the anus and scrotum can induce so much pleasure for our men, but here we are faced with the same prospect again! If my earlier discussion on anilingus wasn't enough to convince your hands to wander in this direction, I certainly hope this will sell you on it! Simply placing a small, firm amount of pressure on this patch will amplify his orgasm tenfold.

Here Comes The Boom

Internally, we know that beyond any reasonable doubt, the longer we can sustain our partner at optimum performance without "pushing him over the edge," the more pleasant his end result will be sooner or later (hopefully *much* later)! Ironically enough, we also know this truth to be somewhat of an oxymoron, as lasting longer in bed requires men to fight their natural, ancestral, inclination to "blow the whistle." To combat this, you can take periodic breaks in the midst of action or to change into some less intense position variations (which comes with transitions breaks inevitably also), to give his overwhelming hormones a chance to recede slightly before hopping back into it. This more than likely will be difficult and require self-discipline especially on his part. Another way to perpetuate when the end is nigh is to place your thumb adamantly on the side of his base, while wrapping your middle and pointer fingers around the circumference and adamantly squeezing just as he is about to burst. Now you're back to square one, and can begin the climb to the summit once more.

"I Just Wanna Feel This Moment"

To be blunt, when seeking to give him the most intense highlight imaginable, there is really one bawdy spot to zone in on: the penis itself. I'm not saying that men don't enjoy touching, kissing, and other sensual spinoff moves, but the bottom line is that when men want to get the most out of the finale, they align themselves into positions that provide the most stimulation **directly**. As mentioned earlier, anal can be beneficial from a standpoint of penetration depth. The vertical nature of the "reverse cowgirl" also provides excellent access for a fast track to the ulterior motive.

"If It Ain't About The Money.."

Whether he's a foreman on a construction crew, or the CEO of a multi-national company, the epic "money shot" has captured the intrigue of men across the board as an ideal element to ice the cake of any sexual interaction. It's interesting that as women, we do not share in this same enthusiasm! According to some of the most popular erotic sites for females, facial porn was listed last on a ranking of most desired sex scenes to least. Despite "facial-finish" having a generally negative stigma in the mass media, it pulls high ratings in the underground world of pornography. We can draw two separate conclusions relating to this. One centers around Darwinian evolution; for instance, since large breasts can be associated healthy levels of estrogen, men may be more inclined toward busty women because that would, in turn, suggest the increased likelihood that they are fertile. The other theory is that because breasts are advertised largely throughout mainstream media, men are essentially brainwashed to focus on this.

The downfall to these theories, is that although they can both be used in justifying different situations, they fail to explain what stems **all** the interests pertaining to sexual fetish found in cult pornography (transgender, grandma, etc). Therefore, we need to consider a third hypothesis: that of erotic dreams. This theory relates more closely to neurological differences between men and women, while also supporting the Darwinian and cultural theory; basically saying that due to the fact that each gender reacts differently to the illusions of the "mind's eye," we can anticipate that the two distinct sexes would have contrasting opinions concerning facials.

For men, specific emotional reactions of women are arousing. We've talked about submissiveness, taking control, being promiscuous, and enthusiastic. But there are others such as innocence. The main point here being:

nothing suggests a woman's emotional reaction better than her face.

You might be asking yourself "how does this all relate to knowing what I should do when he wants to finish *on* me?" The answer is you need to find out what his tastes are and tailor finale to them. Does he find it appeasing to finish on your chin, forehead, cleavage? Or maybe there is a particular phrase he wants to hear you say as added inspiration to prompt the floodgates to open up. I'll leave that portion to you. Believe me, I understand a sticky mess isn't always a girl's dream come true, but I have faith you can tolerate it for his sake.

Epilogue:
Remarks On Non-Verbal
Communication

In the current age of technology and equal rights between men and women, our culture seems almost saturated with political fairness and cross-gender functions. Nevertheless, we still need to acknowledge that there are some very evident differences between us, even down to the molecular level; and these differences absolutely do impact communication.

Our Foundations

The way both sexes deviate through non-verbal communication is a combination of two factors: our upbringing, and our nature. Growing up, I'm sure you heard more than a few of the common idioms that feed into this (think about "cooties," or how "girls can't play sports as well as boys).

"Excuse Me, You're In My Bubble"

It can be interesting to take note of the fact that American men heed larger proximities of personal space than American women. This doesn't carry over to other nationalities necessarily. For example, Arabic men quite frequently walk hand in hand and display other public signs of affection as part of their culture. Furthermore, in western society, women will frequently converse and sit closer to one another than men will. Other trends that have been identified involve violations of personal space (cutting someone off in a line). It has been observed that women are the most probable to fall victim to this.

Read Between the Lines

Comparing the two sexes, women are more emotionally revealing. Men have been socially bred to *internalize*, or hide, what they are feeling when confronted by a catalyst. Perhaps then, it comes as no surprise to learn that women are stronger suited than men in the fields of both actively listening, and deciphering meanings concealed from the plain sight. A female can adjust her style of communicating to the listener more efficiently than a male attempting to do the same.

Body Language

A female typically conveys a wider variety of messages from her smile than a male. Some may include: attraction, shyness, and embarrassment. What about gestures? When I think about a group of guys hanging out, I would expect to see certain cues such as: jock scratching, high-fiving, and fist pumping to project feelings. On the other hand, us women commonly flick our wrists, cross and uncross our legs, and roll our eyes, to place emphasis on what's happening around us.

Conclusion

Well here we are here at last; the end of our rollercoaster ride through the sheets. I hope it was as thrilling for you to read as it was for me to put down on these pages!

The next step is to grab your partner and hit the mattress, tabletop, kitchen sink (if you aren't already!) and put everything outlined here to the test! I know you won't be disappointed!

Finally, if this book effectively helped you as much as I presume, I'd really appreciate it if you spend a few more moments sharing your thoughts over on Amazon.com, so that I can hear all about it.

Happy Humping (wink)!